THE LOW-FODMAP COOKBOOK for BEGINNERS

The Low-FODMAP Diet: A Complete Guide Through a Simple Plan and Many Healthy Recipes to Help Your IBS Relief

TABLE OF CONTENTS

The information in the following pages is broadly considered a truthful and accurate account of facts and as such, any inattention, use, or misuse of the information in question by the reader will render any resulting actions solely under their purview. There are no scenarios in which the publisher or the original author of this work can be in any fashion deemed liable for any hardship or damages that may befall them after undertaking information described herein.

Additionally, the information in the following pages is intended only for informational purposes and should thus be thought of as universal. As befitting its nature, it is presented without assurance regarding its prolonged validity or interim quality. Trademarks that are mentioned are done without written consent and can in no way be considered an endorsement from the trademark holder.

BREAKFAST

Almond Butter Smoothie

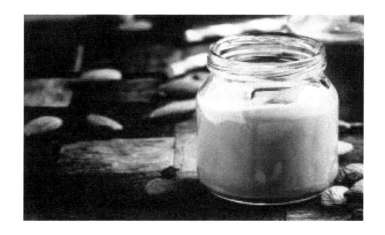

Preparation Time: 5 minutes

Cooking Time: 5 minutes

Servings: 2

INGREDIENTS:

- 3 cups almond milk, unsweetened
- 12 ice cubes
- ¼ Tsp. pure almond extract, sugar-free
- 1 tbsp. ground cinnamon
- ¼ cup flax meal
- 30 drops Stevia sweetener, liquid
- ¼ cup almond butter, unsalted and softened

DIRECTIONS:

1. Combine almond milk, ground cinnamon, flax meal, almond extract, liquid Stevia, ice cubes, and almond butter into a blender.
2. Pulse for 60 seconds or until the consistency is smooth.
3. Divide into two serving cups and enjoy!

NUTRITION: Protein: 14g Carbohydrates: 24g Fat: 24g Sodium: 196g Fiber: 2g Calories: 344

Banana Smoothie

Preparation Time: 5 minutes

Cooking Time: 5 minutes

Servings: 2

INGREDIENTS:

- 2 medium bananas, peeled and sliced
- ¼ Tsp. ground nutmeg
- 1 cup almond milk, unsweetened
- ½ cup gluten-free rolled oats
- 1 Tsp. pure vanilla extract, sugar-free
- ¼ Tsp. ground cinnamon
- 1 Tsp. pure maple syrup
- ¼ cup canned coconut milk, chilled

DIRECTIONS:

1. Open a can of coconut milk and empty out the liquid in a lidded container to use in a different recipe.
2. Use a food blender to pulse maple syrup, nutmeg, cinnamon, vanilla extract, solid coconut milk, oats, almond milk, and bananas for approximately 60 seconds or until it is a smooth consistency.
3. Divide between 2 glasses and enjoy immediately!

NUTRITION: Protein: 15g Carbohydrates: 53g Fat: 5g Sodium: 81g Fiber: 7g Calories: 274

Berry Smoothie

Preparation Time: 5 minutes

Cooking Time: 5 minutes

Servings: 2

INGREDIENTS:

- 1 cup blueberries, Frozen
- 2 cups almond milk, unsweetened
- 2 medium bananas
- ⅛ Tsp. ground cinnamon
- 1 cup strawberries, Frozen

DIRECTIONS:

1. Pulse blueberries, almond milk, bananas, and strawberries in a food blender for approximately 60 seconds or until a smooth consistency.
2. Distribute to 2 glasses and dust with cinnamon. Enjoy immediately!

NUTRITION: Protein: 10g Carbohydrates: 55g Fat: 6g Sodium: 117g Fiber: 6g Calories: 293

Breakfast Wrap

Preparation Time: 5 minutes

Cooking Time: 5 minutes

Servings: 4

INGREDIENTS:

- 4 corn tortillas
- 8 slices cheddar cheese
- 2 cups spinach leaves
- ½ cup avocado

DIRECTIONS:

1. Remove the shell from avocado and mash in a glass dish.
2. Rinse spinach leaves and shake to remove excess water.
3. Arrange tortillas on a flat surface.
4. Evenly divide and layer avocado, spinach leaves, and cheddar cheese on each.
5. Rotate to enclose, starting at the base.
6. Enjoy immediately.

NUTRITION: Protein: 9g Carbohydrates: 15g Fat: 13g Sodium: 156g Fiber: 3g Calories: 205

Cinnamon Almond Crepes

Preparation Time: 10 minutes

Cooking Time: 20 minutes

Servings: 4

INGREDIENTS:

- ½ cup almond flour*
- 2 medium bananas
- ¼ Tsp. pure vanilla extract, sugar-free
- 1 cup almond milk, separated
- ¼ Tsp. ground cinnamon
- 2.67 tbsp. extra virgin olive oil, separated

DIRECTIONS:

1. Empty 2 teaspoons of olive oil into a skillet and allow it to warm up.
2. In the meantime, blend almond milk, bananas, vanilla extract, cinnamon, and almond flour in a glass dish with an electric beater for 45 seconds.
3. Transfer a ladle of batter to the pan and swirl it around to distribute it evenly around.
4. Heat for 30 seconds or until edges turn darker, then turn to the other side.
5. Warm for an additional 30 seconds, then transfer to a serving platter. Enclose with tin foil.
6. Empty another 2 teaspoons in the skillet and repeat steps 3 through 6 until you have completed 8 crepes.

7. Enjoy immediately with your favorite fruits or compote.

NUTRITION: Protein: 3g Carbohydrates: 17g Fat: 11g Sodium: 29g Fiber: 2g Calories: 165

Cranberry Orange Smoothie

Preparation Time: 10 minutes

Cooking Time: 5 minutes

Servings: 2

INGREDIENTS:

- 1⅛ cups orange juice, freshly squeezed
- 1 cup cranberries, raw
- ¼ cup almond milk, unsweetened
- 1 medium banana
- 1 tbsp. lemon juice
- 1 Tsp. pure maple syrup
- 1 cup of ice cubes

DIRECTIONS:

1. Use a glass dish to squeeze orange juice and remove the seeds.
2. Transfer to a food blender and pulse cranberries, almond milk, banana, lemon juice, maple syrup, and ice until it reaches your desired consistency.
3. Divide between two glasses and enjoy immediately!

NUTRITION: Protein: 3g Carbohydrates: 38g Fat: 1g Sodium: 18g Fiber: 4g Calories: 164

French toast

Preparation Time: 10 minutes

Cooking Time: 25 minutes

Servings: 4

INGREDIENTS:

- 1 cup almond milk, unsweetened
- 1⅓ cup tofu, firm and plain
- 2 Tsp. pure vanilla extract, sugar-free
- 4 slices gluten-free bread of your choice
- 4 Tsp. extra virgin olive oil, separated
- 2 tbsp. pure maple syrup

DIRECTIONS:

1. Use a food blender to pulse vanilla extract, almond milk, and tofu until a smooth consistency.
2. Add 2 teaspoons of olive oil into a large skillet and warm.
3. Transfer the wet mix to a shallow dish and immerse the bread in it for 60 seconds on each side. Transfer to a plate until ready to brown.
4. Cook 2 slices at once for 3 minutes on each side, then transfer to a serving platter.
5. Repeat for remaining slices of bread until complete.
6. Top with maple syrup and enjoy while warm.

NUTRITION: Protein: 11g Carbohydrates: 26g Fat: 10g Sodium: 184g Fiber: 1g Calories: 230

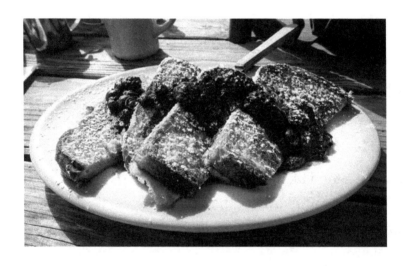

Green Hibiscus Smoothie

Preparation Time: 15 minutes

Cooking Time: 10 minutes

Servings: 2

INGREDIENTS:

- 1 hibiscus tea bag
- ½ inch ginger root, peeled
- ½ cup of water
- 1 cup zucchini, cubed
- ½ cup raspberries, Frozen
- ½ cup of coconut milk, liquid

DIRECTIONS:

1. Empty water into a mug and nuke in the microwave for 1 minute.
2. Insert the tea bag and allow it to steep for 5 minutes.
3. In the meantime, scrub zucchini and chop into small cubes. Transfer to a food blender.
4. Wash raspberries and shake to remove excess water. Transfer to the food blender. Remove
5. Remove tea bag from the water, and empty it into the blender.
6. Combine ginger and coconut milk in the blender and pulse for approximately 30 seconds or until smooth.
7. Transfer to two glasses and enjoy immediately!

NUTRITION: Protein: 2g Carbohydrates: 8g Fat: 12g Sodium: 11g Fiber: 3g Calories: 142

Hearty Oatmeal

Preparation Time: 5 minutes

Cooking Time: 10 minutes

Servings: 4

INGREDIENTS:

- 4 cups of water
- ½ Tsp. iodized salt
- 2 cups gluten-free rolled oats
- ½ Tsp. ground cloves
- 1 Tsp. ground cinnamon
- 4 tbsp. chia seeds
- ½ Tsp. ground nutmeg
- 4 tbsp. pure maple syrup

DIRECTIONS:

1. Empty salt and water into a saucepan and warm on the highest heat setting until it starts to bubble.
2. Combine oats into hot water and heat for 5 minutes while occasionally tossing.
3. Blend ground cloves, chia seeds, ground cinnamon, ground nutmeg, and maple syrup, then warm for another 5 minutes.
4. Serve immediately and enjoy!

NUTRITION: Protein: 8g Carbohydrates: 45g Fat: 3g Sodium: 300g Fiber: 8g Calories: 171

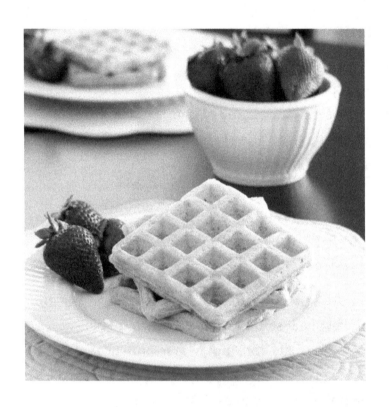

Immune Boosting Smoothie

Preparation Time: 5 minutes

Cooking Time: 10 minutes

Servings: 2

INGREDIENTS:

- 2 cups spinach
- 1-inch ginger root, peeled
- 2 kale leaves
- 2 medium rib celery
- ⅛ Tsp. iodized salt
- 2 medium cucumber
- 2 tbsp. lime juice
- 2 cups ice

DIRECTIONS:

1. Thoroughly rinse spinach, celery, and kale, then shake to remove any extra water. Remove the tough ends of the kale and discard.
2. Scrub cucumbers well and chop into small sections.
3. Use a food blender to pulse salt, lime juice, ginger, cucumbers, celery, kale, and spinach until a smooth consistency.
4. Combine ice and continue to pulse until it reaches your desired consistency.
5. Distribute to two glasses and enjoy it immediately!

NUTRITION: Protein: 3g Carbohydrates: 9g Fat: 1g Sodium: 221g Fiber: 3g Calories: 49

LUNCH

Shrimp with Beans

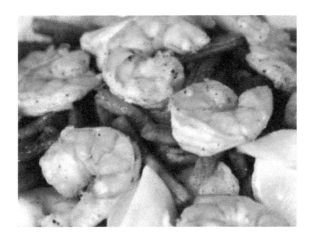

Preparation Time: 10 minutes

Cooking Time: 10 minutes

Servings: 4

INGREDIENTS:

- 1 Lb. shrimp, peeled and deveined
- 2 Tbsp. soy sauce
- ½ Lb. green beans, washed and trimmed
- 2 Tbsp. olive oil
- Salt

DIRECTIONS:

1. Heat oil in a pan.
2. Add beans to the pan and sauté for 5-6 minutes or until tender.
3. Remove pan from heat and set aside.
4. Add shrimp in the same pan and cook for 2-3 minutes each side.
5. Return beans to the pan along with soy sauce. Stir well and cook until shrimp is done.
6. Season with salt and serve.

NUTRITION: Calories: 217, Total Fat: 9g, Saturated Fat: 1.6g, Protein: 27.4g, Carbs: 6.4g, Fiber: 2g, Sugar: 0.9g

Broccoli Fritters

Preparation Time: 10 minutes

Cooking Time: 15 minutes

Servings: 4

INGREDIENTS:

- 3 cups broccoli florets
- 1/3 cup parmesan cheese, grated
- ½ cup flour, gluten-free
- 1 large egg, lightly beaten
- 2 Tbsp. olive oil
- Pepper
- Salt

DIRECTIONS:

1. Steam broccoli florets until tender. Let it cool completely and chop.
2. In a bowl, add egg, cheese, flour, pepper, and salt. Mix well.
3. Add chopped broccoli into the egg mixture and mix well. If the mixture is too dry, then add a tablespoon of water.
4. Heat the olive oil in a pan over medium heat.
5. Make patties from the mixture and cook on the hot pan for 3 minutes each side.
6. Serve and enjoy.

NUTRITION: Calories: 208, Total Fat: 11.6g, Saturated Fat: 3.4g, Protein: 9.1g, Carbs: 16.6g, Fiber: 2.2g, Sugar: 1.3g

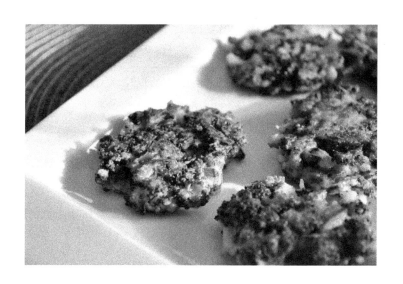

Roasted Broccoli

Preparation Time: 10 minutes

Cooking Time: 15 minutes

Servings: 8

INGREDIENTS:

- 8 cups broccoli florets
- ½ Tsp. Red chili flakes
- 2 Tbsp. soy sauce
- ¼ cup olive oil

DIRECTIONS:

1. Preheat the oven to 425 F
2. Spray a baking tray w/ cooking spray and set aside.
3. Add all of the ingredients to the large mixing bowl and toss well—transfer broccoli mixture on a prepared baking tray.
4. Roast in preheated oven for 15 minutes.
5. Serve and enjoy.

NUTRITION: Calories: 87, Total Fat: 6.6g, Saturated Fat: 0.9g, Protein: 2.8g, Carbs: 6.3g, Fiber: 2.4g, Sugar: 1.6g

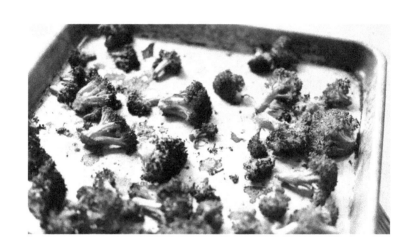

Roasted Maple Carrots

Preparation Time: 10 minutes

Cooking Time: 25 minutes

Servings: 3

INGREDIENTS:

- 1 Lb. baby carrots
- 2 Tsp. Fresh parsley, chopped
- 1 Tbsp. Dijon mustard
- 2 Tbsp. butter, melted
- 3 Tbsp. maple syrup
- Pepper
- Salt

DIRECTIONS:

1. Preheat the oven to 400 o F
2. In a large bowl, toss carrots with Dijon mustard, maple syrup, butter, pepper, and salt.
3. Transfer carrots to baking tray and spread evenly.
4. Roast carrots in preheated oven for 25-30 minutes.
5. Serve and enjoy.

NUTRITION: Calories: 177, Total Fat: 8.1g, Saturated Fat: 4.9g, Protein: 1.3g, Carbs: 26.2g, Fiber: 4.6g, Sugar: 19.2g

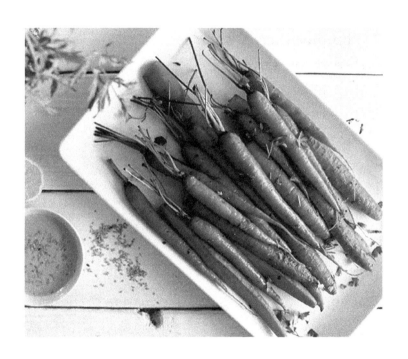

Sweet & Tangy Green Beans

Preparation Time: 10 minutes

Cooking Time: 15 minutes

Servings: 6

INGREDIENTS:

- 1 ½ Lb. green beans, trimmed
- 1 Tbsp. maple syrup
- 2 Tbsp. Dijon mustard
- 2 Tbsp. rice wine vinegar
- ¼ cup olive oil
- ½ cup pecans, chopped
- Pepper
- Salt

DIRECTIONS:

1. Preheat the oven to 400 o F
2. Place pecans on baking tray and toast in preheated oven for 5-8 minutes.
3. Remove from the oven and let it cool.
4. Boil a water in a large pot over high heat.
5. Add green beans in boiling water and cook for 4-5 minutes or until tender. Drain beans well and place in a large bowl.
6. Whisk together oil, maple syrup, mustard, and vinegar in a bowl.

7. Season beans with pepper and salt. Pour oil mixture over green beans.
8. Add pecans and toss well.
9. Serve and enjoy.

NUTRITION: Calories: 139, Total Fat: 10.4g, Saturated Fat: 1.4g, Protein: 2.5g, Carbs: 10.9g, Fiber: 4.3g, Sugar: 3.7g

Sautéed Carrots and Beans

Preparation Time: 10 minutes

Cooking Time: 10 minutes

Servings: 2

INGREDIENTS:

- 2 cups green beans, trimmed
- 1 Tbsp. fresh lemon juice
- 2 Tbsp. butter
- 1 cup baby carrots, halved lengthwise
- 1 Tbsp. olive oil
- Pepper
- Salt

DIRECTIONS:

1. Heat olive oil in a large pan.
2. Add carrots to the pan & cook for a minute.
3. Add green beans and cook until beans are just tender, season with pepper and salt.
4. Once vegetables are cooked, then remove from pan and place on a plate.
5. Turn heat to medium-low and add butter in the same pan. Once butter is melted, then add lemon juice and stir well.
6. Return vegetables to the pan and toss well to coat.
7. Serve and enjoy.

NUTRITION: Calories: 233, Total Fat: 18.7g, Saturated Fat: 8.4g, Protein: 2.2g, Carbs: 16g, Fiber: 6.8g, Sugar: 6.7g

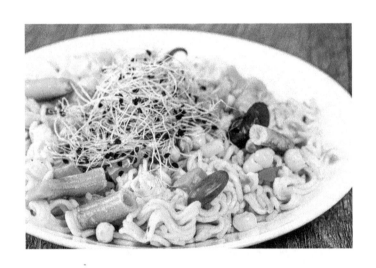

DINNER

Cheeseburger Macaroni

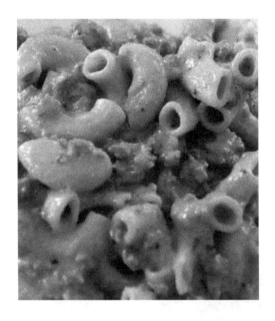

Preparation Time: 10 minutes

Cooking Time: 25 minutes

Servings: 4

INGREDIENTS:

- 1 Lb. ground beef
- 1 cup cheddar cheese, shredded
- 1 Tsp. Chili powder
- 1 ½ Tbsp. prepared mustard
- ¼ cup ketchup
- ½ cup of water
- 14.5 Oz. can tomatoes, diced
- 2 scallions, sliced green part only
- 3 bacon slices, chopped
- 8 Oz. elbow pasta, gluten-free
- ¼ Tsp. Pepper
- ½ Tsp. Salt

DIRECTIONS:

1. Cook macaroni according to packet instructions. Drain well and set aside.
2. Heat large pan over medium heat. Add bacon slices to the pan and sauté until crispy.
3. Add scallions and beef to the pan and sauté until meat is no longer pink.
4. Transfer meat to a paper towel-lined dish to drain grease.

---

5. Add meat, tomatoes, chili powder, mustard, ketchup, water, pepper, and salt into the same pan. Bring to simmer for 5 minutes.
6. Add cheese and cooked macaroni to the pan and cook until cheese is melted about 5 minutes.
7. Serve and enjoy.

NUTRITION: Calories: 659; Total Fat: 24.3g; Saturated Fat: 11.1g; Protein: 55.5g; Carbs: 52.4g; Fiber: 7.5g; Sugar: 8.3g

Salmon Skewers

Preparation Time: 10 minutes

Cooking Time: 10 minutes

Servings: 4

INGREDIENTS:

- 1 Lb. salmon fillets, cut into 1-inch cubes
- 2 Tbsp. soy sauce
- 1 Tbsp. sesame seeds, toasted
- 1 ½ Tbsp. maple syrup
- 1 Tsp. Ginger, crushed
- 1 lime juice
- 1 lime zest
- 2 Tsp. Olive oil

DIRECTIONS:

1. In a bowl, mix together olive oil, soy sauce, lime zest, lime juice, maple syrup, and ginger.
2. Add salmon and stir to coat. Set aside for 10 minutes.
3. Slide marinated salmon pieces onto soaked wooden skewers and grill for 8-10 minutes or until cooked.
4. Sprinkle salmon skewers w/ sesame seeds and serve.

NUTRITION: Calories: 211; Total Fat: 10.5g; Saturated Fat: 1.5g; Protein: 23g; Carbs: 7.4g; Fiber: 0.4g; Sugar: 4.8g

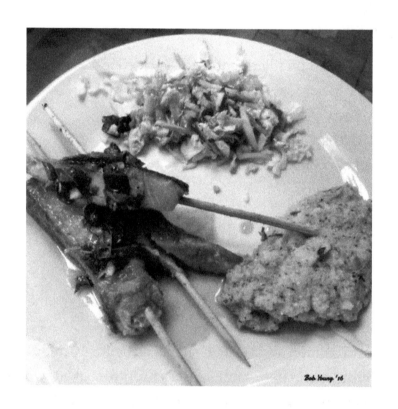

Lemon Chicken

Preparation Time: 10 minutes

Cooking Time: 4 hours

Servings: 4

INGREDIENTS:

- 20 Oz. chicken breasts, skinless, boneless, and cut into pieces
- ¾ cup chicken broth, Low FODMAP
- ½ cup fresh lemon juice
- 1/8 Tsp. Dried thyme
- ¼ Tsp. Dried basil
- ½ Tsp. Dried oregano
- 1 Tsp. Dried parsley
- 2 Tbsp. olive oil
- 2 Tbsp. butter
- 3 Tbsp. rice flour
- 1 Tsp. Salt

DIRECTIONS:

1. In a bowl, toss chicken with rice flour.
2. Heat the butter, and olive oil in a pan over medium-high heat.
3. Add chicken to the pan and cook until brown.
4. Transfer chicken to the slow cooker. Add remaining ingredients on top of chicken.
5. Cover slow cooker w/ lid and cook on low for 4 hours.

6. Serve and enjoy.

NUTRITION: Calories: 423; Total Fat: 23.9g; Saturated Fat: 7.9g; Protein: 42.7g; Carbs: 6.9g; Fiber: 0.4g; Sugar: 0.8g

Dijon Chicken Thighs

Preparation Time: 10 minutes

Cooking Time: 50 minutes

Servings: 4

INGREDIENTS:

- 1 ½ Lb. chicken thighs, skinless and boneless
- 4 Tbsp. maple syrup
- 2 Tsp. Olive oil
- 2 Tbsp. Dijon mustard
- ¼ cup French mustard

DIRECTIONS:

1. Preheat the oven to 375 F/ 190 C.
2. In a mixing bowl, mix together maple syrup, olive oil, Dijon mustard, and French mustard.
3. Add chicken to the bowl & mix until chicken is well coated with maple mixture.
4. Arrange chicken in a baking dish and bake in preheated oven for 45-50 minutes.
5. Serve and enjoy.

NUTRITION: Calories: 401; Total Fat: 15.3g; Saturated Fat: 3.8g; Protein: 49.6g; Carbs: 13.8g; Fiber: 0.3g; Sugar: 12g

Delicious Taco Chicken

Preparation Time: 10 minutes

Cooking Time: 6 hours

Servings: 4

INGREDIENTS:

- 1 Lb. chicken breasts, skinless and boneless
- 1 cup chicken broth, Low FODMAP
- 2 Tbsp. taco seasoning, Low FODMAP

DIRECTIONS:

1. Place chicken in the slow cooker.
2. Mix together chicken broth and taco seasoning and pour over chicken.
3. Cover slow cooker w/ lid and cook on low for 6 hours.
4. Shred the chicken using a fork.
5. Serve and enjoy.

NUTRITION: Calories: 233; Total Fat: 8.7g; Saturated Fat: 2.4g; Protein: 34g; Carbs: 1.7g; Fiber: 0g; Sugar: 0.5g

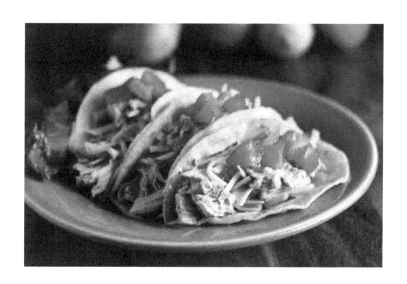

Easy Broiled Fish Fillet

Preparation Time: 10 minutes

Cooking Time: 10 minutes

Servings: 2

INGREDIENTS:

- 2 cod fish fillets
- 2 Tsp. Butter
- ¼ Tsp. Paprika
- 1/8 Tsp. Curry powder
- ½ Tsp. Sugar
- 1/8 Tsp. Pepper
- 1/8 Tsp. Salt

DIRECTIONS:

1. Preheat the broiler.
2. Spray broiler pan w/ cooking spray and set aside.
3. In a small bowl, mix together paprika, curry powder, sugar, pepper, and salt.
4. Coat fish fillet with paprika mixture and place on broiler pan.
5. Broil fish in a preheated broiler for 10-12 minutes or until fish just begins to flakey.
6. Top with butter and serve.

NUTRITION: Calories: 129; Total Fat: 4.9g; Saturated Fat: 2.4g; Protein: 20.1g; Carbs: 1.3g; Fiber: 0.2g; Sugar: 1g

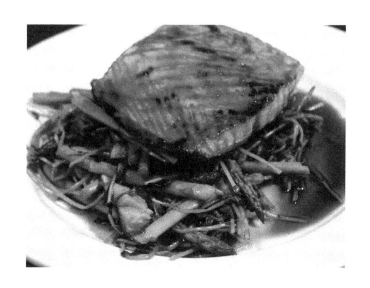

SOUPS RECIPES

Gingered Carrot Soup

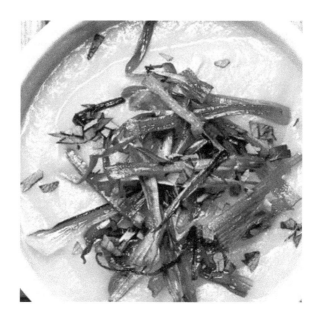

Preparation Time: 5 minutes

Cooking Time: 0 minutes

Servings: 4-6

INGREDIENTS:

- 2 tablespoons butter
- 1 lb. carrots, peeled and diced
- 2 tablespoons fresh grated ginger
- ½ teaspoon salt
- ½ teaspoon black pepper
- ½ teaspoon cinnamon
- ½ teaspoon nutmeg
- 4 cups chicken or vegetable broth (FODMAP compliant)
- 1 cup cooked pumpkin, mashed
- 1 cup almond milk, or other FODMAP compliant milk alternatives
- ¼ cup walnuts, chopped
- ¼ cup fresh parsley, chopped

DIRECTIONS:

1. Add the butter to a large soup pan or stockpot.
2. Once the butter is hot, add in the carrots, salt, black pepper, cinnamon, and nutmeg and sauté, occasionally stirring for 5-7 minutes or until tender.
3. Add the ginger and cook 1-2 additional minutes
4. Add in the broth, & increase the heat to medium-high.
5. Bring the broth to a boil, then reduce the heat to low and simmer for 15 minutes.

6. Add the pumpkin to the soup, and using an immersion blender, blend until creamy. If you don't have an immersion blender, transfer the soup in batches to a traditional blender and puree until creamy.
7. Stir in the almond milk until desired consistency is reached.
8. Continue cooking over low heat for 5 minutes.
9. Serve garnished with fresh parsley and walnuts.

NUTRITION: 253 calories, 121.8 mg calcium, 10.2 g fat, 2 mg iron, 2 g saturates, 16 g sugars, 0.4 g salt, 10.4 g protein, 1.5 g fiber 48 g carbohydrates.

Rustic Potato Soup

Preparation Time: 10 minutes

Cooking Time: 35 minutes

Servings: 6

INGREDIENTS:

- ¼ lb. bacon, diced
- 6 medium-sized potatoes, cut into cubes
- 2 cups carrots, diced
- 3 cups Swiss chard, chopped
- ½ teaspoon salt
- ½ teaspoon black pepper
- 1 teaspoon dried thyme
- ¼ cup fresh parsley
- 2 tablespoons fresh chives
- 5 cups chicken or vegetable broth (FODMAP compliant)
- ½ cup fresh grated parmesan cheese
- ½ cup almond milk, or preferred FODMAP compliant milk alternative

DIRECTIONS:

1. Place the bacon in a large soup pan or stockpot over medium-high heat.
2. Cook the bacon, frequently stirring, until the bacon is browned and crisp.

3. Add the carrots, & cook while stirring for an additional 4-5 minutes.
4. Next, add in the Swiss chard, potatoes, salt, black pepper, and thyme—Cook for 1-2 minutes.
5. Add in the broth & bring the liquid to a boil.
6. Once boiling, reduce the heat to low and simmer for 20 minutes, or until the potatoes and the carrots are tender.
7. Remove half of the soup, working in batches if necessary, and transfer it to a blender. Blend until creamy and then transfer it back into the pot with the rest of the soup.
8. Stir in the parsley, chives, parmesan cheese, and almond milk.
9. Continue cooking over low heat for 5-10 mins. before serving.

NUTRITION: 167 calories, 18 mg calcium, 10.2 g fat, 2.7 mg iron, 7 g saturates, 6 g sugars, 0.4 g salt, 14 g protein, 1.5 g fiber 48 g carbohydrates.

Lemon Ginger Chicken and Rice Soup

Preparation Time: 20 minutes

Cooking Time: 15 minutes

Servings: 4-6

INGREDIENTS:

- 1 tablespoon olive oil
- 4 cups bok choy, shredded
- 2 tablespoons fresh grated ginger
- 1 teaspoon lemon zest
- 2 tablespoons soy sauce
- 2 tablespoons lemon juice
- 4-5 cups chicken broth (FODMAP compliant)
- 2 cups cooked, shredded chicken
- 2 cups cooked basmati rice
- 1 tablespoon fresh chives

DIRECTIONS:

1. Heat olive oil in a soup pan or stockpot.
2. Once the oil is hot, add the bok choy, ginger, and lemon zest. Cook, frequently stirring for 3-4 minutes.
3. Next, add in the lemon juice, soy sauce, and chicken broth. Increase the heat to medium-high and bring the liquid to a low boil.
4. Add in the shredded chicken and cooked rice. Reduce the heat to low and simmer for 10 minutes.

5. Serve garnished with fresh chives.

NUTRITION: 323 calories, 121.8 mg calcium, 10.2 g fat, 2.7 mg iron, 2.2 g saturates, 19.6 g sugars, 0.4 g salt, 10.4 g protein, 1.5 g fiber 46.8 g carbohydrates.

Ginger Soup

Preparation Time: 10 minutes

Cooking time: 20 minutes

Servings: 4

INGREDIENTS:

- 12 carrots, peeled and diced
- 14 oz. can coconut milk
- 2 cups vegetable broth, Low FODMAP
- ½ tsp cinnamon
- 2 fresh rosemary sprigs
- 1 Tbsp. fresh ginger, chopped
- 1 ½ tsp turmeric powder
- 2 Tbsp. olive oil
- ¼ tsp pepper
- ¼ tsp salt

DIRECTION:

1. Preheat the oven to 400°F.
2. Place carrots on baking tray & drizzle with olive oil.
3. Roast carrots in preheated oven for 20 minutes.
4. Transfer roasted carrots in a food processor along with remaining ingredients and process until smooth.
5. Serve and enjoy.

NUTRITION: Calories: 358, Total Fat: 29g, Saturated Fat: 20g, Protein: 6.1g, Carbs: 23.1g, Fiber: 5g, Sugar: 9.4g

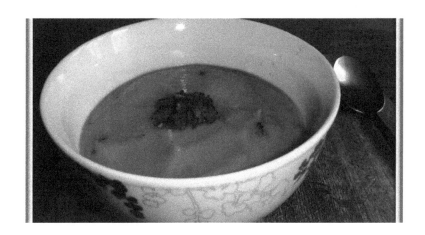

Coconut Zucchini Soup

Preparation Time: 10 minutes

Cooking Time: 28 minutes

Servings: 4

INGREDIENTS:

- 1 zucchini, chopped
- 1 bell pepper, chopped
- 2 carrots, chopped
- 1 cup of coconut milk
- 1 cup of water
- 1 Tbsp. olive oil

DIRECTION:

1. Heat olive oil in a pan over medium heat.
2. Add vegetables to the pan and cook for 7-8 minutes or until they are done.
3. Add coconut milk and stir well—Cook over medium heat for 5 minutes.
4. Add water and cook on low for 15 minutes.
5. Puree the soup using an immersion blender until smooth.
6. Season soup with pepper and salt.
7. Serve and enjoy.

NUTRITION: Calories: 202, Total Fat: 18g, Saturated Fat: 13.2g, Protein: 2.8g, Carbs: 10.8g, Fiber: 3g, Sugar: 5.9g

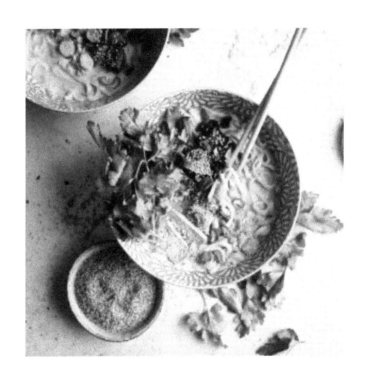

Chicken Noodle Soup

Preparation Time: 5 minutes

Cooking Time: 10 minutes

Servings: 2

INGREDIENTS:

- 2-3 cup of chicken broth
- 2-3 cups of water (fill the container used for broth)
- 1 cup of cooked, chopped chicken breast
- 2-4 oz. of uncooked gluten-free pasta/noodles
- Salt and pepper to taste

DIRECTIONS:

1. Add FODMAP Chicken Broth & Water into a pot.
2. Bring to boil, stirring frequently.
3. Add Uncooked Gluten-Free Pasta & Chicken to the pot.
4. Reduce heat & simmer for around 10 to12 minutes, stirring sporadically.
5. Add Salt & Pepper to taste, if desired.
6. When pasta is cooked to preference, remove from heat.
7. Serve immediately.

NUTRITION: Calories: 109, Total Fat: 15g, Saturated Fat: 10.4g, Protein: 1.5g, Carbs: 6.8g, Fiber: 3g, Sugar: 4.9g

Tomato Carrot Soup

Preparation Time: 10 minutes

Cooking Time: 4 hours

Servings: 4

INGREDIENTS:

- 4 medium carrots, peeled and chopped
- 1 tsp ground cumin
- 1 tsp ground coriander
- 1 Tbsp. turmeric
- 1 cup of coconut milk
- 14.5 oz. can tomatoes, diced

DIRECTION:

1. Add the ingredients into the slow cooker and stir well.
2. Cover slow cooker with lid and cook on low for 4 hours.
3. Puree the soup using an immersion blender until smooth.
4. Serve and enjoy.

NUTRITION: Calories: 193, Total Fat: 14.6g, Saturated Fat: 12.7g, Protein: 3g, Carbs: 15.9g, Fiber: 5g,Sugar: 8.6g

Tomato Basil Soup

Preparation Time: 10 minutes

Cooking Time: 30 minutes

Servings: 4

INGREDIENTS:

- 14 oz. tomato, diced
- 2 tsp coriander
- ½ cup fresh basil, chopped
- ½ cup chicken broth, Low FODMAP
- 21 oz. tomato puree
- 2 ½ cups fennel bulbs, chopped
- 1 ½ Tbsp. butter
- Pepper
- Salt

DIRECTION:

1. Melt the butter in a saucepan over medium heat.
2. Add fennel to the pan and sauté for 10 minutes over medium-high heat.
3. Add tomatoes, coriander, broth, and tomato puree and stir well. Bring to boil then turn heat to low and simmer for 20 minutes.
4. Remove from heat and stir in basil leaves.
5. Season the soup with pepper and salt.
6. Serve and enjoy.

NUTRITION: Calories: 135, Total Fat: 5.1g, Saturated Fat: 2.9g, Protein: 4.8g, Carbs: 21.4g, Fiber: 5.8g, Sugar: 9.9g

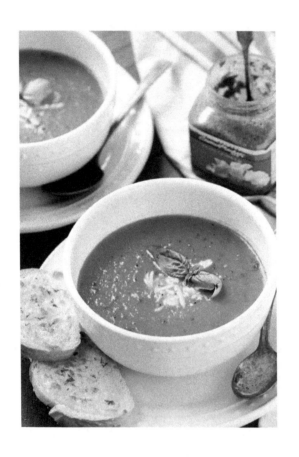

SEAFOOD RECIPES

Dover Sole with Thyme & Parsley Butter

Preparation Time: 10 minutes

Cooking Time: 35 minutes

Servings: 4

INGREDIENTS:

- 4 Dover sole, cleaned and head removed
- 1 Tbsp. fresh thyme
- 1 Tbsp. fresh parsley
- ¼ cup salted butter
- What you'll need from the store cupboard:
- Salt and freshly ground black pepper

DIRECTIONS:

1. Preheat the oven to 375°F.
2. Season the fish w/ salt & freshly ground pepper.
3. Place the fish in a shallow dish & pour in water to around a ¼ inch depth.
4. Bake for 20 to 30 mins. depending on the size of the fish.

5. While the fish is cooking, make the herb butter by melting the butter in a small saucepan. Stir in the herbs.

6. Just before serving, make the herb butter: In a saucepan, gently melt the butter, then stir in freshly chopped herbs.

7. To serve, place the fish and spoon over the herb butter.

NUTRITION: Calories 169, Total Fat 5g, Saturated Fat 4g, Total Carbs 0g, Net Carbs 0g, Sugar 0g, Fiber 0g, Protein 31g, Sodium 6mg.

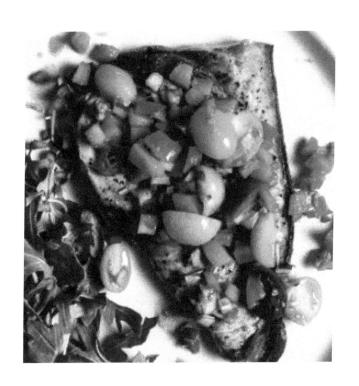

Grilled Swordfish with Tomato Olive Salsa

Preparation Time: 5 minutes

Cooking Time: 8 minutes

Servings: 6

INGREDIENTS:

- 6 5Oz. swordfish steaks, ¾ inch to 1 inch thick
- 2 Tbsp. fresh flat-leaf parsley, chopped
- ½ cup pitted mixed Kalamata and green olives, chopped
- 1½ cup fresh plum tomatoes, cored, seeded and diced
- 2 Tbsp. fresh basil, chopped
- What you'll need from the store cupboard:
- 1 Tbsp. balsamic vinegar
- ½ Tsp. dried basil
- 8 Tbsp. garlic-infused oil
- 2 Tbsp. drained, brined small capers
- Salt and freshly ground black pepper

DIRECTIONS:

1. Combine the chopped tomatoes, 6 tablespoons of oil, olives, 1 tablespoon of basil, capers, and vinegar in a bowl. Season to taste with salt and pepper. Set aside for about one hour to allow the flavors to amalgamate.
2. Make a marinade for the fish by blending the remaining oil and basil and lemon juice in a large bowl. Season with

salt & pepper and allow the fish to marinate for 10 minutes.

3. Set the grill to high & grill the fish for approximately 3-4 minutes on each side.

4. Serve the fish w/ the salsa spooned over the top.

NUTRITION: Calories 331, Total Fat 25g, Saturated Fat 0g, Total Carbs 2g, Net Carbs 2g, Sugar 1g, Fiber 0g,Protein 23g, Sodium 48mg.

Cod with Preserved Lemons & Basil

Preparation Time: 10 minutes

Cooking Time: 10 minutes

Servings: 3

INGREDIENTS:

- 1lb cod loin, cut into 2 pieces
- ⅓ preserved lemon, chopped
- 3 Tbsp. fresh basil leaves, chopped
- 2 Tbsp. fresh parsley, chopped
- What you'll need from the store cupboard:
- 2 Tbsp. garlic-infused oil
- Salt and freshly ground black pepper

DIRECTIONS:

1. Preheat oven to 400°F.
2. Drizzle one tablespoon of the oil on the bottom of a large roasting pan.
3. Place fish in pan and season with salt and pepper: Scatter lemons and two tablespoons of the basil over the fish.
4. Drizzle with remaining oil and bake for approximately 10 minutes.
5. Serve immediately with remaining basil and parsley sprinkled over the top.

NUTRITION: Calories 213, Total Fat 11g, Saturated Fat 0g, Total Carbs 1g, Net Carbs 1g, Sugar 0g, Fiber 0g, Protein 27g, Sodium 586mg.

Chili Coconut Crusted Snapper with Chips

Preparation Time: 15 minutes

Cooking Time: 30 minutes

Servings: 4

INGREDIENTS:

- 1lb Snapper or other mild white fish
- 1 Tbsp. mild green chilies, finely sliced
- 1 Tbsp. fresh lime zest
- 5 cup potato
- ½ cup Colby, cheddar cheese, or soy-free cheese, grated
- What you'll need from the store cupboard:
- 4 Tbsp. sesame oil
- ¼ cup dried shredded coconut
- 1 Tbsp. vegetable oil
- 1 lemon
- Salt & freshly ground black pepper

DIRECTIONS:

1. Leave the shredded coconut to soak in a bowl with water for 10 minutes.
2. Heat half sesame oil in a large skillet and fry the scallions.
3. Add chilies and coconut and fry for one minute. Remove from the pan and set aside.

4. Add the remaining sesame oil to the pan and cook the potatoes until golden in two batches. Season the chips w/ salt and pepper and keep warm.

5. In a separate skillet, fry the fish for 2 minutes on each side in the vegetable oil.

6. Transfer the fish to a shallow baking dish and sprinkle over the cheese and top with coconut crust.

7. Grill the fish for 2 minutes until the crust is brown.

8. Make a basic salad of lettuce, tomatoes, and cucumbers to serve with your fish and chips.

NUTRITION: Calories 486, Total Fat 21g, Saturated Fat 8g, Total Carbs 45g, Net Carbs 37g, Sugar 9g, Fiber 8g, Protein 34g, Sodium 80mg.

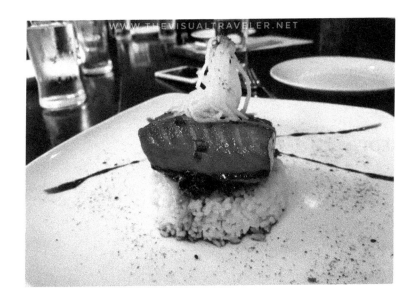

SIDE DISHES, SAUCES AND DIPS RECIPES

Chive and Onion-Infused Dip

Preparation Time: 5 minutes

Cooking Time: 5 minutes

Servings: 10

INGREDIENTS:

- Onion chunks
- 3 tablespoons olive oil
- Mayonnaise
- Parsley, chopped
- Chives, dried
- Lemon juice

DIRECTIONS:

1. Fry the onion in olive oil for 4 minutes.
2. Once fragrant, remove all of the onion chunks from the oil. Set aside to cool.
3. Now place the Ingredients: in a bowl & mix well. Add more lemon juice, parsley, and chives if desired.
4. Refrigerate for 30 minutes.

NUTRITION: Each serving contains 82 calories, 11.9 milligrams calcium, 7.8 grams fat, 0.3 milligrams iron, 1.2 grams saturates, 0.8 grams sugars, 0.2 grams salt, 0.4 grams protein, 0.3 grams of fiber 2.9 grams carbohydrates.

Traditional Hummus

Preparation Time: 10 minutes

Cooking Time: 12 minutes

Servings: 8

INGREDIENTS:

- 400 grams canned chickpeas, rinsed, drained and skinned
- 3 tablespoons water
- 2 tablespoons tahini
- ½ teaspoon salt
- 1 tablespoon olive oil
- 2 tablespoons lemon juice
- ½ teaspoon cumin, ground
- 2 teaspoons garlic-infused oil

DIRECTIONS:

1. Put tahini & lemon juice in a food processor. Blend until smooth.
2. Add remaining ingredients into the tahini mixture. Blend until desired consistency is obtained.
3. Refrigerate for 30 minutes.

NUTRITION: 83 calories, 25.5 milligrams of calcium, 7.9 grams fat, 1-milligram iron, 1.2 grams saturates, 0.2 grams sugars, 0.2 grams salt, 2.3 grams protein, 0.8 grams fiber 1.9 grams carbohydrates.

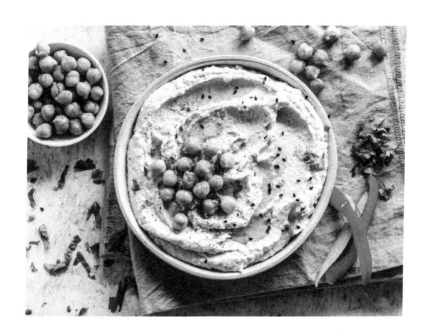

Sunflower Seed Butter

Preparation Time: 15 minutes

Cooking Time: 40 minutes

Servings: 26

INGREDIENTS:

- 40 grams of raw sunflower seeds, hulled
- 1 tablespoon pure maple syrup
- 1 tablespoon coconut oil
- ¼ teaspoon salt

DIRECTIONS:

1. Set the oven to 190 degrees Celsius.
2. Distribute the sunflower seeds evenly on a roasting tray lined with baking paper.
3. Bake for 20 minutes. Stir the seeds every 5 minutes throughout the cook. Set aside to cool.
4. Transfer the seeds to a food processor. Blitz the seeds for 20 minutes. Remember to stop every now and then to scrape the sides of the food processor and break down the lumps in the mixture.
5. Add the remaining Ingredients once butter is creamy and smooth—Blitz for another minute.

NUTRITION: 101 calories, 13.5 milligrams calcium, 8.9 grams fat, 0.9 milligrams iron, 1.2 grams saturates, 1.4 grams of fiber, 3.4 grams protein, 0.9 grams of sugars 3.8 grams of carbohydrates.

Pumpkin and Roast Pepper Hummus

Preparation Time: 10 minutes

Cooking Time: 15 minutes

Servings: 15

INGREDIENTS:

- 200 grams chickpeas, rinsed and drained
- ½ teaspoon cumin, ground
- 1 red bell pepper, deseeded and sliced
- 1 ½ teaspoon paprika
- 400 grams buttercup squash, peeled and sliced
- 3 tablespoons lemon juice
- 2 tablespoons olive oil
- 4 tablespoon water
- 1 tablespoon garlic-infused oil

DIRECTIONS:

1. Set the oven to 190 degrees Celsius.
2. Put bell pepper strips in a tray and sprinkle olive oil on top—roast for 10 minutes.
3. Place squash and water in a bowl. Set microwave on high and heat it while covered for 9 minutes.
4. Now put the remaining ingredients in a food processor. Add squash and bell pepper—season to taste.
5. Blend until smooth.

NUTRITION: 59 calories, 11.9 milligrams calcium, 3.4 grams fat, 0.4 milligrams iron, 0.5 gram saturates, 2.2 grams fiber, 1.6 grams protein, 2.1 grams sugars 6.3 grams carbohydrates.

Pumpkin Dip

Preparation Time: 20 minutes

Cooking Time: 40 minutes

Servings: 8

INGREDIENTS:

- 500 grams buttercup squash, peeled and sliced
- ½ tablespoon garlic-infused oil
- 1 tablespoon canola oil
- 2 tablespoons lemon juice
- 2 tablespoons mayonnaise
- ½ teaspoon paprika
- 1 tablespoon fresh rosemary, chopped
- Salt and pepper

DIRECTIONS:

1. Set the oven to 200 degrees Celsius.
2. Put pumpkin pieces in a tray and drizzle with oil— season to taste.
3. Roast for 30 minutes then set aside for 10 minutes to cool.
4. Transfer the roast pumpkin to a food processor. Add remaining ingredients and blend until smooth.

NUTRITION: 58 calories, 10.6 milligrams calcium, 3.8 grams fat, 0.3 milligrams iron, 0.5 grams saturates, 2.7 grams sugars, 0.1 gram salt, 1.3 grams protein, 2.6 grams fiber 6.2 grams carbohydrates.

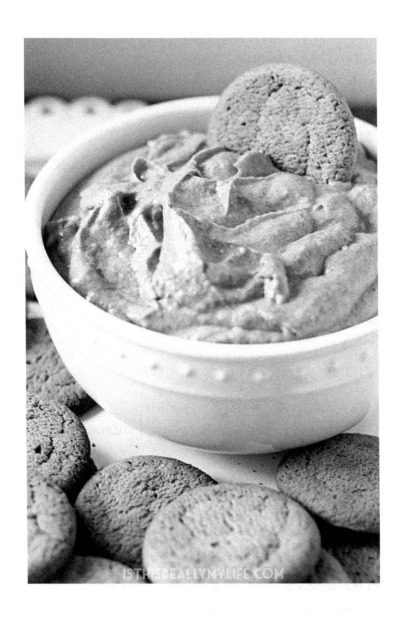

SNACKS, DESSERT AND APPETIZER RECIPES

Millet Chocolate Pudding

Preparation Time: 10 minutes

Cooking Time: 0 minutes

Servings: 4

INGREDIENTS:

- 1 Lb. cooked millet
- 2 cup unsweetened almond milk
- ½ medium banana
- ¼ cup of cocoa powder
- 2 tablespoons maple syrup
- What you'll need from the store cupboard:
- None

DIRECTIONS:

1. Pour all ingredients in a blender and then pulse until smooth.
2. Pour the chocolate mixture into bowls and allow to set in the fridge before serving.

NUTRITION: Calories 260, Total Fat 5.8g, Saturated Fat 2.9g, Total Carbs 45.9g, Net Carbs 42.4g, Protein 8.9g, Sugar: 14.3g, Fiber: 3.5g, Sodium: 27mg, Potassium: 443mg

Vanilla Maple Chia Pudding

Preparation Time: 10 minutes

Cooking Time: 0 minutes

Servings: 1

INGREDIENTS:

- 3 tablespoons chia seeds
- 1 cup of coconut milk
- ½ teaspoon vanilla extract
- 1 tablespoon maple syrup
- What you'll need from the store cupboard:
- None

DIRECTIONS:

1. Mix all ingredients in a container and stir until well combined.
2. Place inside the fridge and allow to set overnight.

NUTRITION: Calories 280, Total Fat 12.6g, Saturated Fat 5.1g, Total Carbs 31.7g, Net Carbs 26.5g, Protein 10.2g, Sugar: 24.2g, Fiber: 5.2g, Sodium: 110mg, Potassium: 452mg

Dark Chocolate Gelato

Preparation Time: 10 minutes

Cooking Time: 10 minutes

Servings: 16

INGREDIENTS:

- 2 ¼ cups of coconut milk
- ¾ cup lactose-free heavy cream
- 2 tablespoons arrowroot starch
- ½ cup of cocoa powder
- 4 Oz. dark chocolate
- What you'll need from the store cupboard:
- ¾ cup of sugar

DIRECTIONS:

1. In a saucepan, place half of the coconut milk, cream, arrowroot starch, cocoa powder, and dark chocolate. Add in the sugar.
2. Turn on the stove & bring the mixture to a simmer until it thickens. Turn off the heat and add the remaining milk. Mix until well combined.
3. Pour into an ice cream maker. Turn the ice cream maker for 3 hours until the mixture turns into a gelato.
4. If you do not have an ice cream maker, you can place the mixture in a lidded container. Place in the fridge for 8 hrs. But make sure that you mix the mixture every hour to create the creamy gelato texture.

NUTRITION: Calories 145, Total Fat 11.4g, Saturated Fat 9.1g, Total Carbs 11g, Net Carbs 7.5g, Protein 2.5g, Sugar: 3.4g, Fiber: 3.5g, Sodium: 20mg, Potassium: 299mg

Bread Pudding with Blueberries

Preparation Time: 10 minutes

Cooking Time: 40 minutes

Servings: 2

INGREDIENTS:

- 1 extra-large egg
- 2/3 cup unsweetened almond milk
- 1 tablespoon maple syrup
- ¼ teaspoon vanilla extract
- 4 slices of gluten-free bread
- ½ cup blueberries
- A dash of ground cinnamon
- What you'll need from the store cupboard:
- None

DIRECTIONS:

1. Preheat the oven to 3750F.
2. In a bowl, almond milk, whisk the eggs, and maple syrup until well combined. Add in the vanilla extract.
3. Cut the crusts from the bread & slice the bread into tiny cubes. Place the bread cubes in a greased baking dish and pour the egg mixture. Top with blueberries and sprinkle with a dash of cinnamon.
4. Bake for 40 minutes or until the egg mixture is set and the top has browned and puffed up.

NUTRITION: Calories 268, Total Fat 6.5g, Saturated Fat 2.6g, Total Carbs 44.9g, Net Carbs 42.8g, Protein 7.8g, Sugar: 25.6g, Fiber: 2.1g, Sodium: 238mg, Potassium: 215mg

Chocolate English Custard Recipes

Preparation Time: 10 minutes

Cooking Time: 10 minutes

Servings: 2

INGREDIENTS:

- 1 ½ tablespoon tapioca starch
- 1 egg
- 1 tablespoon pure maple syrup
- ¾ cup almond milk
- 1 tablespoon water
- 1 ½ tablespoon cocoa powder
- What you'll need from the store cupboard:
- None

DIRECTIONS:

1. Add all ingredients in a saucepan and whisk until all lumps are removed.
2. Place the saucepan on the stove and then bring to a boil over low heat while stirring constantly.
3. Turn off the heat once the mixture thickens.
4. Pour into ramekins and refrigerate for 3 hours before serving.

NUTRITION: Calories 170, Total Fat 6.5g, Saturated Fat 2.1g, Total Carbs 24.6g, Net Carbs 21.4g, Protein 5.8g, Sugar: 16.2g, Fiber: 3.2g, Sodium: 340mg, Potassium: 892mg

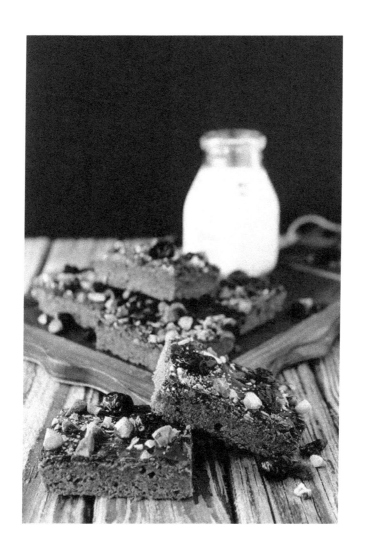

DRINKS

Warm Ginger Tea

Preparation Time: 5 minutes

Cooking Time: 0 minutes

Servings: 1

INGREDIENTS:

- 1 cup boiling water
- 2" piece fresh ginger root, grated
- Juice of 1/2 medium lemon
- 1 teaspoon pure maple syrup
- 1/4 teaspoon freshly ground black pepper
- 1/4 teaspoon Himalayan salt

DIRECTIONS:

1. Pour water into a teacup and add all Ingredients. Let sit for 2–3 minutes.

NUTRITION: Calories: 27 Fat: 0g Protein: 0g Sodium: 597mg Fiber: 1g Carbohydrates: 8g Sugar: 5g

Ginger Maple Tea

Preparation Time: 5 minutes

Cooking Time: 0 minutes

Servings: 1

INGREDIENTS:

- 1 cup of water
- 1 teaspoon freshly grated ginger root
- 2 slices lemon
- 1 teaspoon ground cinnamon
- 1 tablespoon maple syrup

DIRECTIONS:

1. Boil water and pour 3⁄4 into a mug. Add ginger, lemon, cinnamon, and maple syrup and allow to steep 10 minutes.
2. Add remaining 1⁄4 cup boiling water. Relax and sip slowly.

NUTRITION: Calories: 68 Fat: 0g Protein: 0g Sodium: 10mg Fiber: 2g Carbohydrates: 18g Sugar: 12g

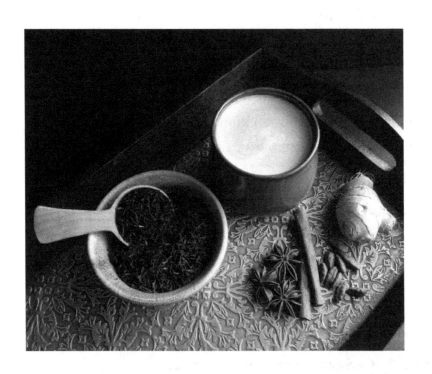

Aloe Vera Rewind

Got acid reflux, constipation, or ulcerative colitis? This drink may help, as it contains aloe and turmeric, which have both been known to help fight inflammation.

Preparation Time: 5 minutes

Cooking Time: 0 minutes

Servings: 1

INGREDIENTS:

- 2 tablespoons aloe Vera gel
- 1/2 cup chopped cucumber
- Juice of 1 medium lime
- 8 ounces cold water
- 1/4 teaspoon ground turmeric

DIRECTIONS:

1. Place all ingredients in a blender. Blend well and add to glass. Cover glass with plastic wrap and chill in refrigerator 1 hour before consuming.

NUTRITION: Calories: 30 Fat: 0g Protein: 1g Sodium: 9mg Fiber: 2g Carbohydrates: 9g Sugar: 2g

Blueberry Ginger Water

This refreshing drink will complement a day in the shade and it's great when you want something other than water.

Preparation Time: 5 minutes

Cooking Time: 0 minutes

Servings: 2

INGREDIENTS:

- Makes 1 cup
- 1 cup coarsely chopped gingerroot, unpeeled
- 1 cup turbinate sugar
- 3 cups of water
- 1 tablespoon lime juice (per serving)
- 1/4 cup blueberries (per serving)

DIRECTIONS:

1. Place ginger in a food processor & process until rough in texture.
2. Place ginger, sugar, and water in a medium saucepan. Bring to a boil, then reduce heat to low and simmer; cook 1 hour or until liquid has reduced to 1 cup of glossy liquid.
3. Place a sieve over a medium bowl—strain syrup through a sieve, pushing gently down on ginger. Allow syrup to cool slightly before storing in a glass bottle or jar. Before

using refrigerate for several hours or overnight. Keep refrigerated 2–3 weeks.

4. Once you're ready to use the syrup, measure 1 tablespoon into an 8-ounce glass with water and ice. Add lime juice and blueberries. Enjoy!

NUTRITION: Calories: 858 Fat: 3g Protein: 6g Sodium: 96mg Fiber: 11g Carbohydrates: 212g Sugar: 200g

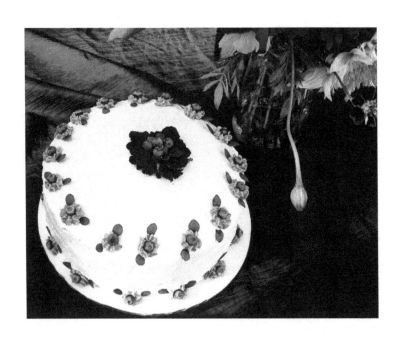

Blue Moon Smoothie

For those who love blueberries and chia seeds, this smoothie is a true fit.

Preparation Time: 5 minutes

Cooking Time: 0 minutes

Servings: 1

INGREDIENTS:

- 1⁄2 cup unsweetened coconut milk
- 10 frozen blueberries
- 1⁄2 ripe medium banana
- 1 tablespoon chia seeds
- 1 cup crushed ice

DIRECTIONS:

1. Place milk in a blender followed by other Ingredients & blend until smooth. Add more milk or ice if desired. Enjoy!

NUTRITION: Calories: 289 Fat: 24g Protein: 3g Sodium: 16mg Fiber: 2g Carbohydrates: 20g Sugar: 10g

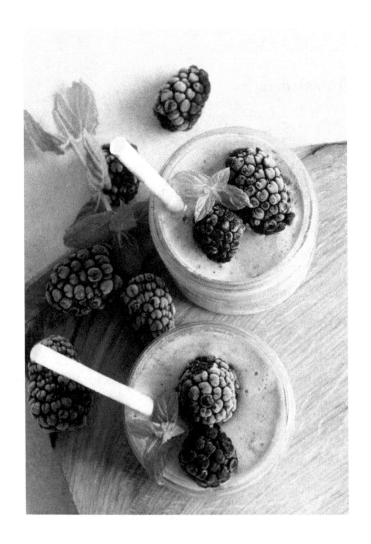

Shamrock Shake

Try this smoothie and top o' the morning to you and your day!

Preparation Time: 5 minutes

Cooking Time: 0 minutes

Servings: 1

INGREDIENTS:

- 1⁄2 cup lactose-free milk
- 1⁄2 frozen ripe medium banana
- 1⁄8 medium avocado
- 1–2 leaves romaine lettuce or a handful of baby spinach
- 1⁄4 teaspoon alcohol-free vanilla extract
- 1⁄8 teaspoon alcohol-free peppermint extract

DIRECTIONS:

1. Place milk in a blender first followed by a 1⁄2 cup ice and remaining ingredients and blend until smooth. Add more milk or add ice if desired. Enjoy!

NUTRITION: Calories: 158 Fat: 5g Protein: 6g Sodium: 60mg Fiber: 4g Carbohydrates: 24g Sugar: 15g

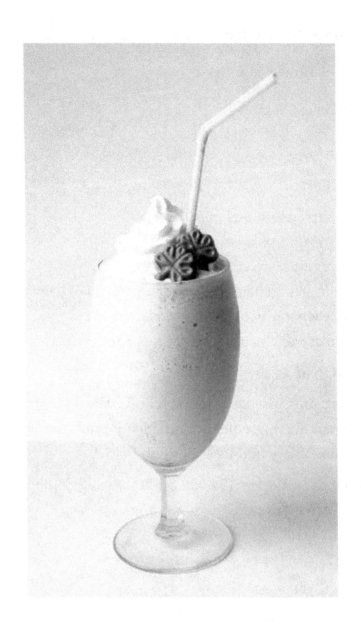

CPSIA information can be obtained
at www.ICGtesting.com
Printed in the USA
BVHW091543190421
605296BV00003B/344

9 781802 331790